D1372912

Contents

Introduction

This healthy elimination diet plan helps identify food intolerances and sensitivities to alleviate digestive issues or other common symptoms.

People may start an elimination diet for several reasons, with one of the main reasons being to try and pinpoint food intolerances and sensitivities that cause digestive issues like gas, bloating or stomach pain. A food intolerance is where your body processes a certain food (or foods) in a different way than others, which can cause that gastrointestinal discomfort or other symptoms. Food intolerances are different from a food allergy, which involves an immune response that can be very dangerous. If you suspect a true food allergy, we encourage you to discuss this with your medical provider or allergist.

In this elimination diet plan, we map out a week of meals and snacks that include delicious flavors and easy recipes. What didn't we include? The top 8 foods most commonly associated with food intolerances, sensitivities and food allergies milk, eggs, tree nuts, peanuts, wheat, soy, fish and shellfish. We set this plan at 1,500 calories a day but included modifications to make it 1,200 calories or 2,000 calories, depending on your needs.

Food intolerances and sensitivities are extremely common. In fact, it's estimated that between 2–20% of people worldwide may suffer from a food intolerance. Elimination diets are the gold standard for identifying food intolerances, sensitivities and allergies through diet.

They remove certain foods known to cause uncomfortable symptoms and reintroduce them at a later time while testing for symptoms. Allergists and registered dietitians have been using elimination diets for decades to help people rule out foods that are not tolerated well.

What Is an Elimination Diet?

A food elimination diet is a systematic approach used to identify food sensitivities. Food elimination diets can take on a number of different forms. In this plan, we excluded foods that contain the 8 most common allergens, but if you strongly suspect that, for example, dairy is the culprit and choose to only replace dairy items with nondairy alternatives, you can modify this plan as needed.

There's also something called the low-FODMAP diet, which is most often used to help people diagnosed with irritable bowel syndrome. The low-FODMAP diet limits certain types of carbohydrates that can cause gastrointestinal distress in those with IBS. which is where this meal plan can come in handy. You can use this plan as a guide and template for what to eat (or not to eat) and adjust it according to your individual needs.

After the designated elimination phase, the next phase is reintroduction, where you introduce one possible food trigger back into your diet at a time. You should space out these reintroductions by at least three days, so it's easier to determine what trigger foods cause what symptoms. It can be very helpful to keep a food symptoms diary during this time. This means you'll keep track of what you eat as well as what symptoms you're having and when.

An elimination diet involves removing foods from your diet that you suspect your body can't tolerate well. The foods are later reintroduced, one at a time, while you look for symptoms that show a reaction. It only lasts 5–6 weeks and is used to help those with a sensitive gut, food intolerance or food allergy identify which foods are contributing to their symptoms.

In that way, an elimination diet may alleviate symptoms like bloating, gas, diarrhea, constipation and nausea. Once you have successfully identified a food your body can't tolerate well, you can remove it from your diet to prevent any uncomfortable symptoms in the future.

There are many types of elimination diets, which all involve eating or removing certain types of foods. However, if you have a known or suspected food allergy, then you should only try an elimination diet under the supervision of a medical professional. Reintroducing a food allergen may trigger a dangerous condition called anaphylaxis.

If you suspect you have a food allergy, check with your doctor before starting an elimination diet. Symptoms of an allergy include rashes, hives, swelling and difficulty breathing.

Elimination diets pretty much do exactly what the name suggests: exclude certain foods for a short period of time usually 3 weeks. Then you slowly reintroduce specific foods and monitor your symptoms for possible reactions.

An elimination diet involves removing foods from your diet that you suspect your body can't tolerate well. The foods are later reintroduced, one at a time, while you look for symptoms that show a reaction. It only lasts 5–6 weeks and is used to help those with a sensitive gut, food intolerance or food allergy identify which foods are contributing to their symptoms. In that way, an elimination diet may alleviate symptoms like bloating, gas, diarrhea, constipation and nausea.

Once you have successfully identified a food your body can't tolerate well, you can remove it from your diet to prevent any uncomfortable symptoms in the future. There are many types of elimination diets, which all involve eating or removing certain types of foods. However, if you have a known or suspected food allergy, then you should only try an elimination diet under the supervision of a medical professional.

Reintroducing a food allergen may trigger a dangerous condition called anaphylaxis. If you suspect you have a food allergy, check with your doctor before starting an elimination diet. Symptoms of an allergy include rashes, hives, swelling and difficulty breathing.

How to Do an Elimination Diet and Why

Food intolerances and sensitivities are extremely common. In fact, it's estimated that between 2–20% of people worldwide may suffer from a food intolerance. Elimination diets are the gold standard for identifying food intolerances, sensitivities and allergies through diet.

They remove certain foods known to cause uncomfortable symptoms and reintroduce them at a later time while testing for symptoms. Allergists and registered dietitians have been using elimination diets for decades to help people rule out foods that are not tolerated well.

Why Do An Elimination Diet?

Elimination diets are used to identify food sensitivities and intolerances. Elimination diets work a lot like a science experiment to help you identify foods that lead to a wide range of bothersome symptoms.

Types Of Elimination Diets

In this article, we've included a food list for one type of elimination diet, but many other elimination diets exist. They include:

The Whole Foods Elimination Diet

Highly-processed foods house a wide range of additives that can trigger gut irritation and sensitivities in many people. These include food colorings, sugar alcohols, monosodium glutamate (MSG), and sulfites, among others.

By shifting to a diet rich in minimally-processed whole foods, you can naturally reduce or eliminate those food chemicals while boosting your overall health. As an added bonus, minimally-processed whole foods tend to contain fiber and other nutrients that nourish the digestive tract.

- Eliminate just 1 food or food category

If you're pretty sure you already know which food causes your problems, this is a great option. Let's say, for example, from past experience, you know that you feel pretty horrid whenever you eat dairy. Then, on this type of elimination diet, you'd eliminate just dairy for 3 weeks. Then you'd reintroduce it to see how you feel.

- Eliminate up to 4 foods

This is another great option if you're pretty sure you know what foods bother you. To do it, only eliminate 1-4 foods that you think might cause problems for you.

The Precision Nutrition Elimination Diet

We usually refer to this as the "elimination diet medium" because it offers a middle way between hardly removing anything at all and removing so many foods that you think you can't last another day. You'll find a food list a little later in this story that shows you, in detail, which foods to eat and which foods to remove.

The Full Elimination Diet

This much more extensive type of elimination diet excludes a wide range of foods, including many types of meat, legumes, grains, nuts, and seeds even a wide variety of fruits and veggies.

Because of the highly-restrictive nature of this elimination diet, however, you should only try it with the guidance of a professional who specializes in integrative medicine and/or medical nutrition therapy.

The FODMAP Elimination Diet

FODMAP stands for:

- Fermentable
- Oligosaccharides
- Disaccharides
- Monosaccharides
- Polyols

These carbohydrate fibers are not fully absorbed in the small intestine. For many people, that's not an issue. But in people with Irritable Bowel Syndrome (IBS), this incomplete digestion can trigger a range of bothersome symptoms: gas, distension, pain, diarrhea, and/or constipation.Over several years, researchers at Monash University in Australia have developed and extensively studied a low-FODMAP elimination diet for people with IBS, showing that it can help to alleviate these symptoms.

Unlike other types of elimination diets, however, the FODMAP diet is a highly specialized form of medical nutrition therapy. The reintroduction phase of this diet is much more complex than the reintroduction phase of a typical elimination diet.

As a result, if you've been diagnosed with IBS and suspect you might have a FODMAP issue, you'll need the expertise of someone qualified to offer medical nutrition therapy, such as a FODMAP-trained nutritionist.

How Does It Work?

- The Elimination Phase

The elimination phase involves removing foods you suspect trigger your symptoms for a short period of time, typically 2–3 weeks. Eliminate foods that you think your body can't tolerate, as well as foods that are notorious for causing uncomfortable symptoms. Some of these foods include nuts, corn, soy, dairy, citrus fruits, nightshade vegetables, wheat, foods containing gluten, pork, eggs and seafood .

During this phase, you can determine if your symptoms are due to foods or something else. If your symptoms still remain after removing the foods for 2–3 weeks, it is best to notify your doctor.

- The Reintroduction Phase

The next phase is the reintroduction phase, in which you slowly bring eliminated foods back into your diet. Each food group should be introduced individually, over 2–3 days, while looking for symptoms. Some symptoms to watch for include:

- Rashes and skin changes
- Joint pain
- Headaches or migraines
- Fatigue
- Difficulty sleeping
- Changes in breathing
- Bloating
- Stomach pain or cramps
- Changes in bowel habits

If you experience no symptoms during the period where you reintroduce a food group, you can assume that it is fine to eat and move on to the next food group.

However, if you experience negative symptoms like those mentioned above, then you have successfully identified a trigger food and should remove it from your diet. The entire process, including elimination, takes roughly 5–6 weeks.

If you plan to eliminate many food groups, seek advice from your doctor or a dietitian. Eliminating too many food groups may cause a nutritional deficiency.

What's A Food Sensitivity? What's A Food Intolerance?

According to the American Academy of Allergy Asthma & Immunology, "A food intolerance or a food sensitivity occurs when a person has difficulty digesting a particular food."

Unlike food allergies which involve the immune system food sensitivities occur when the gut reacts poorly to specific foods and ingredients. These reactions generally unfold in a couple ways:

- Inflammation: Certain foods irritate gut tissues, leading to symptoms throughout the body. For example, the amines naturally present in red wine can expand blood vessels, triggering migraines in some people.
- Indigestion: Other times, the digestive tract fails to properly break down certain foods. For example, you've probably heard of lactose intolerance. Some people's

intestines don't produce enough of the enzyme lactase to digest lactose, a sugar present in dairy. The result: gas, bloating, and diarrhea.

What Symptoms Can Be Addressed By An Elimination Diet?

A growing body of evidence shows that food sensitivities can lead to a wide range of unwanted symptoms.[1,2] For example, food sensitivities have been linked to:

- Bloating
- Brain fog
- Depression
- Diarrhea
- Fatigue
- Headaches
- Obesity
- Pain[1]
- Rashes
- Stomach aches

And much more.

You may wonder: If food sensitivities involve the gut, how do symptoms show up all over the body in the skin (rashes), brain (headaches), or joints (pain)? Here's why. Our gastrointestinal (GI) tract does a lot more than just digest and absorb food. Surprisingly, the GI tract also has its own independently working nervous system (aka the enteric nervous system).

Therefore, the GI tract is rich in neurotransmitters, hormones, chemical messengers, enzymes, and bacteria. Indeed, it's even home to 70 percent of your body's entire immune system.Food sensitivities may also contribute, directly or indirectly, to many other problematic aspects of digestion: microbial imbalances, motility issues, detoxification abnormalities, and intestinal permeability.

This explains why problems in the gut can show up all over in the form of migraines, chronic pain, eczema and other rashes, and brain fog, among many other symptoms and health problems. So it makes sense that, if you're suffering from food sensitivities, following an elimination diet for a few weeks could be the most profound dietary change you'll ever make. For some people, the results can feel nothing short of miraculous.

What Are The Benefits Of An Elimination Diet?

Elimination diets help you to collect and analyze empirical evidence, using experimentation and observation based on what happens in your body as you change what you eat. If your headaches disappear after you've removed certain foods only to suddenly resurface when you reintroduce chocolate, that's a powerful clue.

Without an elimination diet, you can only guess about causes and their effects. Are you bloated because of the onions you ate at lunch? Or was it the beer? Or is the bloat from something non-food related, such as eating too quickly?

This guesswork gets even more difficult when:

Symptoms show up outside of the gut. Did you wake with a migraine because of the wine you had with dinner? Or are you just dehydrated? Or maybe you didn't sleep well? Similarly, was that skin rash caused by something you ate or was it caused by contact with a perfume, detergent, or some other irritating substance?

You can eat small amounts of certain foods without symptoms. For example, one square of chocolate might not cause problems, but when you eat half a bar? Your body rebels. Symptoms are delayed. You eat some red pepper and feel fine. Then days later, your joints are achy and swollen. Yep, it's possible. An elimination diet helps you pinpoint the true source of such problems, once and for all.

Elimination Diet Foods List

The foods to avoid on an elimination diet are very individualized. Some people may want to start by avoiding lactose, the carbohydrate found in some dairy products, as it's the most common food intolerance. Other people suspect gluten, the protein in wheat, may cause their symptoms. In this plan, we excluded the top 8 foods most commonly associated with food intolerances, sensitivities and allergens. See the full list of what to avoid with each allergen here.

Milk, including dairy products like yogurt, kefir, butter, cheese, cottage cheese, creamer, half-and-half, sour cream, ice cream, whey or dairy-based powders, any packaged products made with dairy and more. Eggs, including foods made with eggs like some mayonnaise brands, baked goods, egg-based powders and more.

Tree nuts, including almonds, walnuts, pistachios, cashews, pecans, pralines, pine nuts, nut butters, nut milks, nut extracts or pastes and more. Peanuts, including peanut butter, peanut oil, peanut flour and more. Wheat, including wheat-based bread, cereal, pasta, breadcrumbs, crackers, flours and more, bulgur, farro, matzoh meal, seitan, wheatgrass, wheat germ oil and more.

Soy, including soy sauce and tamari, edamame, tofu, tempeh, miso, soymilk, soy yogurt, soy ice cream, soy oil and more.

Fish, including salmon, tuna (fresh or canned), tilapia, bass, anchovies, sardines, haddock, pollock, swordfish, trout and more.

Shellfish, including crabs, crawfish, lobster, shrimp, prawns, clams, mussels, oysters, scallops and more.

What You Can Eat

While you may end up cutting out quite a lot of foods during an elimination diet, there are still so many delicious items you do get to eat! Here are just some of the delicious foods you'll find in this meal plan.

- Fruits & veggies and plenty of them!
- Healthy proteins like beans, chicken and steak.
- Seeds to snack on in place of nuts, like pumpkin seeds and sunflower butter.
- Wheat-free grains, like quinoa, oatmeal and corn tortillas.
- And plenty of herbs and spices to keep your meals flavorful and exciting.

Although an elimination diet is very restricting, there is still enough variety to make healthy and delicious meals. Some foods you can eat include:

- Fruits: Most fruits, excluding citrus fruits.
- Vegetables: Most vegetables, excluding nightshades.
- Grains: Including rice and buckwheat.
- Meat and fish: Including turkey, lamb, wild game and cold-water fish like salmon.
- Dairy substitutes: Including coconut milk and unsweetened rice milk.
- Fats: Including cold-pressed olive oil, flaxseed oil and coconut oil.
- Beverages: Water and herbal teas.

Spices, condiments and others: Including black pepper, fresh herbs and spices (excluding cayenne pepper and paprika) and apple cider vinegar.

To stay motivated during this restrictive phase, try designing new recipes and experimenting with herbs and spices to add delicious flavor to your dishes.

How to Meal-Prep Your Week of Meals

Here's how you can prep ahead for the busy week:

Prepare Meal-Prep Vegan Moroccan Lettuce Wraps to have for lunch on days 2 through 5.

✓ Day 1

Breakfast (322 calories) :

- 1 serving Berry-Coconut Smoothie
- A.M. Snack (131 calories)
- 1 large pear

Lunch (360 calories):

- 1 serving White Bean & Veggie Salad
- P.M. Snack (125 calories)
- 1 medium apple
- 2 tsp. pumpkin seeds

Dinner (540 calories):

- 1 serving Spiced Grilled Chicken with Cauliflower "Rice" Tabbouleh
- 1 serving Cucumber & Avocado Salad

Daily Totals: 1,479 calories, 54 g protein, 167 g carbohydrate, 41 g fiber, 75 g fat, 1,172 mg sodium

How to make it 1,200 calories: Switch to 1 medium orange instead of a pear at A.M. snack, and don't have the Cucumber & Avocado Salad with dinner.

How to make it 2,000 calories: Add 1 1/2 cups unsweetened coconut milk yogurt to A.M. snack, increase to 1/4 cup pumpkin seeds at P.M. snack, and increase to 2 servings Cucumber & Avocado Salad at dinner.

✓ Day 2

Breakfast (322 calories):

- 1 serving Berry-Coconut Smoothie
- A.M. Snack (180 calories)
- 1/4 cup pumpkin seeds

Lunch (425 calories)

- 1 serving Meal-Prep Vegan Moroccan Lettuce Wraps
- P.M. Snack (50 calories)
- 2 oz. deli turkey

Dinner (542 calories)

- 1 serving Roasted Vegetable & Black Bean Tacos

- 1 serving Cucumber & Avocado Salad

Daily Totals: 1,520 calories, 53 g protein, 167 g carbohydrate, 41 g fiber, 80 g fat, 1,769 mg sodium

How to make it 1,200 calories: Switch to 1 clementine instead of pumpkin seeds at A.M. snack, and don't have the Cucumber & Avocado Salad with dinner.

How to make it 2,000 calories: Add 1 large banana to A.M. snack, add 15 gluten-free crackers to P.M. snack, and increase to 2 servings Cucumber & Avocado Salad at dinner.

✓ Day 3

Breakfast (261 calories):

- 1 serving Old-Fashioned Oatmeal
- 1/4 cup blueberries
- 2 Tbsp. pumpkin seeds
- A.M. Snack (105 calories)
- 1 medium banana

Lunch (425 calories):

- 1 serving Meal-Prep Vegan Moroccan Lettuce Wraps
- P.M. Snack (292 calories)
- 1 medium apple

- 2 Tbsp. sunflower butter

Dinner (422 calories):

- 1 serving Braised Chicken Thighs with Olive, Orange & Fennel
- 1/2 cup cooked quinoa

Daily Totals: 1,506 calories, 65 g protein, 177 g carbohydrate, 35 g fiber, 66 g fat, 1,246 mg sodium

How to make it 1,200 calories: Switch to 1 clementine instead of a banana at A.M. snack, and switch to 1 medium orange and don't include the sunflower butter at P.M. snack.

How to make it 2,000 calories: Increase to 1/4 cup pumpkin seeds at breakfast, add 2 Tbsp. sunflower butter at A.M. snack, add 1 medium banana to lunch, and increase to 1 cup cooked quinoa at dinner.

✓ Day 4

Break fast:

- A.M. Snack (131 calories)
- 1 large pear

Lunch (425 calories):

- 1 serving Meal-Prep Vegan Moroccan Lettuce Wraps
- P.M. Snack (180 calories)
- 1/4 cup pumpkin seeds

Dinner (503 calories) :

- 1 serving Chickpea & Quinoa Buddha Bowl

Daily Totals: 1,501 calories, 52 g protein, 198 g carbohydrate, 45 g fiber, 64 g fat, 1,282 mg sodium

How to make it 1,200 calories: Switch to 1/4 cup sliced cucumber at A.M. snack instead of a pear, and replace the pumpkin seeds at P.M. snack with 1/4 cup blueberries.

✓ Day 5

Breakfast (322 calories):

- 1 serving Berry-Coconut Smoothie
- A.M. Snack (275 calories)
- 1 medium apple
- 1/4 cup pumpkin seeds

Lunch (425 calories):

- 1 serving Meal-Prep Vegan Moroccan Lettuce Wraps

- P.M. Snack (50 calories)
- 2 oz. deli turkey

Dinner (450 calories):

- 1 serving Mediterranean Cabbage Soup
- 1 serving Guacamole Chopped Salad

Meal-Prep Tip: Reserve 2 servings of the Mediterranean Cabbage Soup to have for lunch on Days 6 and 7. Daily Totals: 1,522 calories, 53 g protein, 182 g carbohydrate, 47 g fiber, 73 g fat, 1,733 mg sodium

How to make it 1,200 calories: Have 1/2 cup sliced cucumber instead the apple and pumpkin seeds at A.M. snack, and switch to 1/4 cup blueberries instead of deli turkey at P.M. snack.

How to make it 2,000 calories: Add 1 medium orange to lunch, and add 1 large banana with 3 Tbsp. sunflower butter to P.M. snack.

✓ Day 6

Breakfast (322 calories) :

- 1 serving Berry-Coconut Smoothie
- A.M. Snack (275 calories)

- 1 medium apple
- 1/4 cup pumpkin seeds

Lunch (310 calories):

- 1 serving Mediterranean Cabbage Soup
- 1 medium banana
- P.M. Snack (131 calories)
- 1 large pear

Dinner (447 calories):

- 1 serving Grilled Chicken Taco Salad

Daily Totals: 1,485 calories, 57 g protein, 204 g carbohydrate, 41 g fiber, 58 g fat, 1,011 mg sodium

How to make it 1,200 calories: Don't have the pumpkin seeds at A.M. snack, and switch to 1 clementine instead of a pear at P.M. snack.

How to make it 2,000 calories: Add 10 gluten-free crackers with 1 1/2 Tbsp. sunflower butter to P.M. snack, and add 1/4 cup guacamole with 1 oz. corn tortilla chips to dinner.

✓ Day 7

Breakfast (261 calories):

- 1 serving Old-Fashioned Oatmeal
- 1/4 cup blueberries
- 2 Tbsp. pumpkin seeds
- A.M. Snack (302 calories)
- 1 medium banana
- 2 Tbsp. sunflower butter

Lunch (310 calories):

- 1 serving Mediterranean Cabbage Soup
- 1 medium banana
- P.M. Snack (131 calories)
- 1 large pear

Dinner (495 calories):

1 serving Sheet-Pan Steak Fajitas

Daily Totals: 1,500 calories, 62 g protein, 197 g carbohydrate, 39 g fiber, 59 g fat, 1,085 mg sodium

How to make it 1,200 calories: Don't have the sunflower butter at A.M. snack, and switch to 1 clementine instead of a pear at P.M. snack.

How to make it 2,000 calories: Add 1 serving Berry-Coconut Smoothie to breakfast and add 1/4 cup pumpkin seeds to P.M. snack

How to Do an Elimination Diet

If you're wondering how to start an elimination diet, we would first recommend that you meet with a registered dietitian who can help safely guide you through the process. They will discuss your current diet and symptoms and help you think about what your possible food triggers may be. Then, they will likely advise you to completely avoid those trigger foods for at least two weeks, which is where this meal plan can come in handy. You can use this plan as a guide and template for what to eat (or not to eat) and adjust it according to your individual needs.

After the designated elimination phase, the next phase is reintroduction, where you introduce one possible food trigger back into your diet at a time. You should space out these reintroductions by at least three days, so it's easier to determine what trigger foods cause what symptoms. It can be very helpful to keep a food symptoms diary during this time. This means you'll keep track of what you eat as well as what symptoms you're having and when.

How Does An Elimination Diet Work?

Elimination diets are organized into three phases: A prep phase, removal phase, and reintroduction phase.

Prep Phase (7-9 Days)

During the prep phase, you'll have to prepare for the removal phase. This may be the most important part of the diet so don't skip it. People who spend a week getting prepared do far better than people that jump right into it.

Some of your prep work involves keeping a food journal to help identify trigger foods as well as deciding which foods to stop eating during the removal phase. This will help to personalize the elimination diet. This prep time also involves planning what you will eat: finding recipes, finding groceries, organizing your kitchen, and so on.

Removal Phase (3 Weeks)

This is when you stop eating a variety of common trigger foods, such as gluten, dairy, and eggs.

Phase 3: Reintroduction Phase (3+ Weeks)

Now it's time to systematically reintroduce the eliminated foods—testing them one at a time while monitoring for possible reactions.

The Removal Phase: What To Expect

During the removal phase of an elimination diet, you stop eating 1 or more foods. Depending on how many foods you eliminate, you might begin to feel better pretty quickly. Within days to weeks, you might notice clearer skin, heightened energy, more regular bowel movements, improved sleep, and other improvements.

Though this is an encouraging outcome, it's not always evidence that the removal phase is working. For example, more whole foods, fewer highly processed foods, and smaller portions can also lead to improved energy, fewer GI symptoms, and an overall sense of well being.

You won't know for sure whether you have a food sensitivity until you get to the reintroduction phase. Also, it's important to note that not everyone feels better right away.

Some people feel worse before they start to feel better as they withdraw from caffeine, sugar, and other foods.

Foods To Eliminate During The Removal Phase

The following table gives an example of what to include and exclude during a typical elimination diet.

You'll of course find other lists available on the Internet allowing more, and sometimes fewer, foods in the diet. The key here is to not get too dogmatic. Self-experimentation rules the day. Try different things and see what works for you.

Foods to Remove:

- Vegetables Highly-processed veggies (ex: battered and fried)
- Nightshades: eggplant, peppers, tomatoes, white potatoes
- Fruit Dried fruit (with sugar), canned fruit
- Starches Gluten-containing grains: barley, bulgur, couscous, farro, kamut, rye, spelt, triticale, wheat
- Gluten-containing bread, cereal, crackers, pasta, and wraps (including bran pellets, couscous, muesli, orzo, naan, roti)
- Oats*
- Corn
- Legumes Soybeans and soybean products: edamame, miso, natto, soy sauce, soy milk, tempeh, textured vegetable protein, tofu

- Peanuts, peanut butter
- Meat, fish, meat substitutes, & shellfish Eggs
- Processed fish: smoked, canned, and breaded options, such as canned tuna and fish sticks
- Processed meat: bacon, burger patties, canned meats, cold cut, cured sausage, deli meats, hot dogs
- Beef
- Soy-based meat substitutes and seitan
- Dairy & dairy alternatives Milk: cow, oat, goat
- Buttermilk, cheese, condensed milk, cottage cheese, cream, ice cream, custard, non-dairy creamers, sour cream, yogurt
- Fats & oils Butter, dips, canola oil, margarine, mayonnaise, processed and hydrogenated oils, spreads, salad dressings (unless made from oils on the Foods to Eat list)
- Beverages Alcohol: beer, coolers, hard beverages, mixed drinks, spirts, wine
- Caffeinated beverages: black tea, coffee, green tea, energy drinks, soft drinks
- Fruit juice
- Spices & condiments Barbecue sauce, caviar, cayenne pepper, chocolate, chutney, cream-based sauces, curry paste, ketchup, mustard, pasta sauce, paprika, relish, soy sauce, tomato-based sauces, tzatziki

- Sweeteners Brown sugar, corn syrup, coconut sugar, desserts, high fructose corn syrup, honey, jam, maple syrup, raw cane sugar, white sugar

Foods to keep :

- Vegetables: All fresh, raw, steamed, sauteed, or roasted vegetables (except eggplant, tomatoes, peppers, and white potatoes)
- Fruits: All fresh or frozen fruit without added sugar
- Starches: Gluten-free grains: amaranth, brown rice, buckwheat, millet, quinoa, sorghum, teff
- Roots and tubers: beets, parsnip, rutabaga, squash, sweet potato, taro, turnips, yuca
- Legumes: Beans & lentils
- Nuts and seed:
- Tree nuts: almonds, brazil nuts, cashews, hazelnuts, pecans, pistachios, walnuts
- Seeds: chia seeds, flaxseeds, hemp seeds, pinenuts, pumpkin seeds, sesame seeds, sunflower seeds
- Oils & nut butters made from tree nuts, seeds
- Meat, fish, meat substitutes, & shellfish: Meat: chicken, duck, lamb, pork, turkey, wild game
- Fresh fish, shellfish
- Rice-based protein powder

- Dairy & dairy alternatives: Unsweetened coconut, rice, almond, and hemp milk
- Fats and oil: Oils: avocado oil, coconut butter, coconut oil, cold-pressed olive oil, flaxseed oil, grapeseed oil, sesame oil
- Foods: coconut meat, flakes, and milk (unsweetened), olives, avocado.
- Beverages: Water, non-caffeinated herbal teas, mineral water
- Spices and condiments: Apple cider vinegar (and other vinegars without sugar or flavorings)
- Sea salt
- Most fresh herbs and spices (see exceptions in red list)
- Sweeteners: Stevia (if needed)

Removal Phase Meal Ideas

An easy way to adapt to an elimination diet? Make a list of the foods and meals you eat regularly and then look for ways to adapt them. For example, if you plan to follow our Elimination Diet Medium food list above, perhaps you could. Make tacos or burritos in a bowl or lettuce wrap with turkey or tilapia, brown rice, and guac.

Try homemade 100% salmon, lamb, chicken, or bison burgers, either wrapped in lettuce or with sweet potato toast, or eaten on their own.Have pasta made from zucchini noodles or brown rice pasta, mixed with a sauce made from lemon, salt, pepper, and olive oil. Top with roasted salmon.

Add avocado to a smoothie to replace the creaminess of yogurt. Another great strategy is to make a list of all of the foods you can eat, and organize them into these categories: Proteins, vegetables, carbs, healthy fats.

Then, whenever you want to assemble a quick meal, just pick one option from each of those four categories. In other words, you might choose salmon for your protein, broccoli for your veggie, brown rice for your carb, and avocado oil for your fat. Then you might use the oil to roast the broccoli and salmon, serving both with the brown rice. Add herbs and spices as needed.

(Find an extensive Create-a-Meal template, along with additional recipes and food lists, see our new Elimination Diet ebook for nutrition coaches. Download it here. It's free.)

Removal Phase Packaged Food List
Elimination diets can feel pretty restrictive, mostly because so many packaged foods contain gluten, dairy, soy, and corn. To

make this easy, we read label after label, searching for packaged foods that work well with a typical elimination diet removal phase. You'll find a complete packaged food list in our free Elimination Diet ebook for coaches.

Removal Phase Recipes

The following recipes all work with the Elimination Diet food list presented in this story.

- Simple Fruit Smoothie

Blend (in this order): 2 cups coconut or rice milk, 2-4 thumbs of avocado, 2 cupped hands of fruit chunks (use frozen for a thicker smoothie), 2 scoops rice protein powder. (Makes 2 servings.)

- Sweet Potato Toast

Slice a large sweet potato in half lengthwise. Then slice 2 pieces from that center cut on each side, 1/4 " to " thick. Toast until fork tender. (This may take several rounds in a toaster). Alternatively, lightly brush both sides with oil and bake at 350°F for 15-20 minutes, until fork tender, but not soft. Serve topped with ½ mashed avocado, 2 sliced radishes, and sea salt. (Makes 2 servings.)

- Basic energy balls

Blend 10-12 pitted, coarsely chopped dates, 1 cup unsweetened shredded coconut (or any variety of finely chopped nuts, except peanuts), and ½ teaspoon cinnamon in the food processor. Then roll into balls. (Makes about 8 balls, 2 per serving.)

- Avocado cakes

Mash ½ avocado. Spread on 8 Lundberg "Thin Stackers" brown rice cakes. Sprinkle with sea salt. Top each with 1-2 cucumber slices and a small sprig of dill, parsley, or cilantro. (Makes 2 servings.)

- Banana "nice" cream

Coarsely slice 4 ripe bananas into small chunks, set on a plate or baking sheet, and freeze 1-2 hours. Once frozen, add banana chunks to a food processor and blend until creamy, scraping down the sides as necessary. Freeze for 1-2 hours for scoopable ice cream—or eat right away for "soft serve." Top as desired. (Makes 4 servings.)

- Baked Salmon with Brussels Sprouts

On a foil-lined or nonstick baking sheet, combine 1 pound (4 cups) trimmed and halved Brussels sprouts, 2 Tbsp melted coconut oil, 1 cup fresh cranberries, ½ tsp sea salt, and ¼ tsp apple cider vinegar. Scoot to one side of the sheet, then add six 4-oz salmon fillets, seasoned with salt and pepper. Bake at 400°F for 20 minutes, or until the salmon flakes with a fork and the sprouts are golden. (Makes 4 servings.)

The Reintroduction Phase: What To Expect

Of course, it's not the purpose of the elimination diet to get rid of all the foods above forever. That would be awful. Rather, the point is to eliminate the foods and then slowly reintroduce them, one at a time, so you can monitor yourself for symptoms.

During the entire reintroduction phase, pay attention to how you're feeling. For example, you'll want to monitor your sleep, mood, energy, digestion, bowel habits, and so on.

Reintroduce foods using a 3-day cycle:

- Day 1: Reintroduce one food, eating at least two servings of it at different times of the day. For example, clients might reintroduce eggs on a Monday by having two scrambled eggs at breakfast and two hard boiled eggs at lunch.

- Days 2 & 3: Stop eating the new food. For example, if you reintroduce eggs on day 1, you'll stop eating eggs.

- Day 4 and beyond: What happens after day 4 will depend on how things went on days 2 and 3.

If you feel great, you'll reintroduce a different food (say wheat) for one day, repeating the three day cycle.

If you're still experiencing reactions, you'll wait until those symptoms subside before reintroducing another food.

What to do next: By now you should realize that the elimination diet isn't necessarily easy. But it's not that hard either. It just requires that you have a plan and you pay attention.

To get started on an elimination diet, you might want to:

- Download our comprehensive Elimination Diet book for nutrition coaches, which includes food lists, recipes, and all of the resources you or a client would need to get started and be successful.
- Keep a food journal for a few weeks. Jot down what you eat and drink, along with how you feel. Then examine it for clues to see if you can get a sense of the foods leading to your symptoms.
- Try to see this journey as an experiment that helps you learn more about yourself, your body, and your eating choices.
- Consult with your health care provider to learn how such a diet might interact with any health conditions or medicines you might be taking.
- If you decide to give an elimination diet a try, we hope it helps you get to the bottom of your symptoms, learn more about the foods that do and don't work for you, and feel a whole lot better.

What Can't You Eat on an Elimination Diet?

The best elimination diets are the most restricting. The more foods you remove during the elimination phase, the more likely it is that you will discover which foods trigger uncomfortable symptoms.

Foods that are commonly removed during the elimination phase include:

- Citrus fruits: Avoid citrus fruits, such as oranges and grapefruits.
- Nightshade vegetables: Avoid nightshades, including tomatoes, peppers, eggplant, white potatoes, cayenne pepper and paprika.
- Nuts and seeds: Eliminate all nuts and seeds.
- Legumes: Eliminate all legumes, such as beans, lentils, peas and soy-based products.
- Starchy foods: Avoid wheat, barley, corn, spelt, rye, oats and bread. Also avoid any other gluten-containing foods.
- Meat and fish: Avoid processed meats, cold cuts, beef, chicken, pork, eggs and shellfish.
- Dairy products: Eliminate all dairy, including milk, cheese, yogurt and ice cream.
- Fats: Avoid butter, margarine, hydrogenated oils, mayonnaise and spreads.
- Beverages: Avoid alcohol, coffee, black tea, soda and other sources of caffeine.
- Spices and condiments: Avoid sauces, relish and mustard.
- Sugar and sweets: Avoid sugar (white and brown), honey, maple syrup, corn syrup and high-fructose corn syrup, agave nectar, desserts and chocolate.

If you suspect that other foods not on this list make you feel uncomfortable, it is highly recommended to remove them as well.

What Are The Most Common Food Sensitivities?

Based on data we've gathered from the thousands of clients we've coached, we can say pretty confidently that the following categories tend to cause the most problems:

- Gluten
- Dairy
- Eggs
- Sweeteners (example: sugar)
- Soy

Other Types of Elimination Diets

Besides the traditional elimination diet described above, there are several other types of elimination diets. Here are a few different types of elimination diets:

- Low-FODMAPs diet

Removes FODMAPs, which are short-chain carbohydrates that some people can't digest. Few foods elimination diet: Involves eating a combination of foods that you don't eat regularly. One example is the lamb and pears diet, which is popular in the US, where lamb and pears are not commonly eaten.

- Rare foods elimination diet

Similar to a few foods diet, but you can only eat foods that you rarely ever eat, as they are less likely to trigger your symptoms. Common foods on a rare food diet include yams, buckwheat and starfruit.

- Fasting elimination diet

Involves strictly drinking water for up to five days, then reintroducing food groups. This type of diet should only be done with permission from your doctor, as it can be dangerous to your health.

Other elimination diets: These include lactose-free, sugar-free, gluten-free and wheat-free diets, among others.

Benefits of an Elimination Diet

Elimination diets help you discover which foods cause uncomfortable symptoms so you can remove them from your diet.

However, an elimination diet has many other benefits, including:

- It May Reduce Symptoms of Irritable Bowel Syndrome

Irritable bowel syndrome (IBS) is a very common gut disorder that affects between 10–15% of people worldwide.Many people find that an elimination diet improves IBS symptoms like bloating, stomach cramps and gas.

In one study, 150 people with IBS followed either an elimination diet that excluded trigger foods or a fake elimination diet that excluded the same number of foods but not ones linked with uncomfortable symptoms. People who followed the actual elimination diet reduced their symptoms by 10%, and those who best stuck to the diet reduced symptoms by up to 26% .

- It May Help People With Eosinophilic Esophagitis

Eosinophilic esophagitis (EE) is a chronic condition where allergies trigger inflammation of the esophagus, the tube that delivers food from mouth to stomach. People with EE have difficulty swallowing foods that are dry and dense, increasing their risk of choking.

Many studies have shown that elimination diets are effective for improving symptoms of EE .

In one study of 146 patients with EE, over 75% of all patients experienced significantly fewer symptoms and less inflammation through an elimination diet.

- It May Reduce Symptoms of ADHD

ADHD (attention-deficit/hyperactivity disorder) is a behavioral disorder that affects 3–5% of all children and adults.

Studies have shown elimination diets may reduce symptoms of ADHD.One analysis looked at 20 studies that restricted certain foods to improve ADHD symptoms. Researchers found that elimination diets helped reduce ADHD symptoms among children who were sensitive to foods.

However, children should not follow an elimination diet unless supervised by a medical professional. Elimination diets restrict many essential nutrients that are important for growing children, and long-term restriction could stunt their growth.

- It May Improve Skin Conditions Like Eczema

Eczema is a group of skin conditions that appear as red, itchy, cracked and inflamed skin. There are many different causes of eczema, but many people find that eating certain foods can worsen their symptoms.

Several studies have found that elimination diets may reduce symptoms of eczema.In one study of 15 participants with eczema, 14 found that an elimination diet reduced their symptoms and helped identify their trigger foods.

- It May Reduce Chronic Migraines

Roughly 2–3 million people in the US alone suffer from chronic migraines .The causes of migraines are still unclear, but studies have shown that inflammation could be a trigger.

An elimination diet removes foods that cause inflammation and has been shown to reduce chronic migraines. In one study, 28 women and two men with frequent migraines followed an elimination diet for six weeks, which helped reduce the number of headache attacks during that time from nine to six .

What Are The Side Effects Of An Elimination Diet?

Whenever you dramatically change your diet, your body is likely to have a few things to say about it and this can be especially true with elimination diets. Though some people truly feel amazing pretty quickly, other people feel worse before they feel better.

Why? An elimination diet involves a rapid and dramatic change. It's like jumping into high-intensity-interval-training after being out of shape for years. This is especially true if you go from a heavy intake of caffeine, sugar, and highly-processed foods to a zero intake of these foods and beverages.

As a result, you may initially notice withdrawal symptoms like headaches, fatigue, irritability, or skin flare-ups for a few days to a week. This healthy elimination diet plan helps identify food intolerances and sensitivities to alleviate digestive issues or other common symptoms.

People may start an elimination diet for several reasons, with one of the main reasons being to try and pinpoint food intolerances and sensitivities that cause digestive issues like gas, bloating or stomach pain. A food intolerance is where your body processes a certain food (or foods) in a different way than others, which can cause that gastrointestinal discomfort or other symptoms.

Food intolerances are different from a food allergy, which involves an immune response that can be very dangerous. If you suspect a true food allergy, we encourage you to discuss this with your medical provider or allergist.

In this elimination diet plan, we map out a week of meals and snacks that include delicious flavors and easy recipes. What didn't we include? The top 8 foods most commonly associated with food intolerances, sensitivities and food allergies milk, eggs, tree nuts, peanuts, wheat, soy, fish and shellfish. We set this plan at 1,500 calories a day but included modifications to make it 1,200 calories or 2,000 calories, depending on your needs.

Risks of an Elimination Diet

Although elimination diets are a great way to discover which foods cause you problems, they also come with a few risks. For starters, elimination diets should only be followed for a short period of time, or between four and eight weeks.

Following an elimination diet for longer is not recommended, as it could cause nutrient deficiencies as a result of eliminating certain food groups. Additionally, children and people with known or suspected allergies should only do an elimination diet under the supervision of a doctor.

Because elimination diets are restricting, taking away certain food groups for even a short period of time could stunt a child's growth.Children are also more prone to severe reactions, like anaphylaxis, when reintroducing a food group. This is because their bodies can become extra sensitive to foods after avoiding them.

Conclusion

A good elimination diet is very restricting, which helps you identify as many trigger foods as possibleElimination diets can reduce the intake of important nutrients if followed for too long. Children and people with known or suspected allergies should not follow an elimination diet unless supervised by their doctor.

Elimination diets can help you determine which foods your body can't tolerate well. If you're experiencing symptoms that you think may be related to your diet, then an elimination diet could help you discover which foods are causing them.

However, elimination diets are not for everyone. Children should not try an elimination diet unless supervised by a doctor or dietitian. Likewise, people with known or suspected allergies should only try an elimination diet the under the supervision of a doctor. Finally, it's important to note that elimination diets should only be done short-term, as long-term restrictions may cause nutritional deficiencies.

An elimination diet is a short-term diet that helps identify foods your body can't tolerate well and removes them from your diet. An elimination diet works by removing foods you think cause discomfort. It then reintroduces them individually to check for symptoms.

Although elimination diets are restricting, there are still plenty of food options to make healthy and delicious meals. There are many different types of elimination diets, including the low-FODMAPs diet, the few foods diet, the rare foods diet, fasting and more. An elimination diet may benefit people with IBS, ADHD, migraines, eosinophilic esophagitis and skin conditions like eczema.

Made in the USA
Middletown, DE
03 December 2023

44426651R00031